This
Beauty Journal
Belongs to

_____

_____

DEDICATION

This Beauty Journal book is dedicated to all the glamorous and elegant people out there who love to try new products, log their daily beauty routines, and document their findings in the process.

You are my inspiration for producing books and I'm honored to be a part of keeping all of your Beauty notes and records organized.

This journal notebook will help you record your details about your beauty process.

Thoughtfully put together with these sections to record: MakeUp Inventory, Hair Products Inventory, Skincare Products Inventory, Beauty Wish List, Product Reviews, My Beauty Recipes, and Daily Beauty Journal Pages.

HOW TO USE THIS BOOK:

The purpose of this book is to keep all of your Beauty notes all in one place. It will help keep you organized.

This Beauty Journal will allow you to accurately document every detail about trying and reviewing new products and recording your daily routine. It's a great way to chart your course through glamorous beautification.

Here are examples of the prompts for you to fill in and write about your experience in this book:

1. MakeUp Inventory - Item, Brand, Price, Rating.

2. Hair Products Inventory - Item, Brand, Price, Rating.

3. Skincare Products Inventory - Item, Brand, Price, Rating.

4. Beauty Wish List - List all the products you want to try (Makeup, Skin Care, Body & Hair, Tools).

5. Product Reviews - Review any products, listing all the important information, plus notes for an overall review.

6. My Beauty Recipes - Name of Recipe, Used For, Ingredients, How To Make.

7. Daily Beauty Journal Pages - Date, Beauty Steps, Hair & Body Care, I Feel Beautiful Today Because, Sleep Tracker, Water Intake Tracker.

Enjoy!

Make Up Inventory

Item	Brand	Price	Rating 1-5

Make Up Inventory

Item	Brand	Price	Rating 1-5

Hair Products Inventory

Item	Brand	Price	Rating 1-5

Hair Products Inventory

Item	Brand	Price	Rating 1-5

Skin Products Inventory

Item	Brand	Price	Rating 1-5

Skin Products Inventory

Item	Brand	Price	Rating 1-5

Beauty Wishlist

Make Up	Skin Care	Body & Hair	Tools

Beauty Wishlist

Make Up	Skin Care	Body & Hair	Tools

Beauty Wishlist

Make Up	Skin Care	Body & Hair	Tools

Beauty Wishlist

Make Up	Skin Care	Body & Hair	Tools

Product Reviews

Item: _____

Brand: _____   Price: _____
                        Purchase Date: _____
Purchase Place: _____
Expiration Date: _____
Purchase Again: YES   NO
INGREDIENTS: _____
_____

Overall Review: _____
_____
_____
_____
_____

Item: _____

Brand: _____   Price: _____
                        Purchase Date: _____
Purchase Place: _____
Expiration Date: _____
Purchase Again: YES   NO
INGREDIENTS: _____
_____

Overall Review: _____
_____
_____
_____

Product Reviews

Item: _____

Brand: _____ Price: _____
                       Purchase Date: _____

Purchase Place: _____

Expiration Date: _____

Purchase Again: YES   NO

INGREDIENTS: _____

_____

Overall Review: _____

_____

_____

_____

Item: _____

Brand: _____ Price: _____
                       Purchase Date: _____

Purchase Place: _____

Expiration Date: _____

Purchase Again: YES   NO

INGREDIENTS: _____

_____

Overall Review: _____

_____

_____

_____

Product Reviews

Item:

Brand: Price:
                                Purchase Date:

Purchase Place:

Expiration Date:

Purchase Again: YES   NO

INGREDIENTS:

Overall Review:

Item:

Brand: Price:
                                Purchase Date:

Purchase Place:

Expiration Date:

Purchase Again: YES   NO

INGREDIENTS:

Overall Review:

Product Reviews

Item:

Brand: Price:
                                Purchase Date:

Purchase Place:

Expiration Date:

Purchase Again: YES   NO

INGREDIENTS:

Overall Review:

Item:

Brand: Price:
                                Purchase Date:

Purchase Place:

Expiration Date:

Purchase Again: YES   NO

INGREDIENTS:

Overall Review:

Product Reviews

Item:

Brand: Price:

Purchase Date:

Purchase Place:

Expiration Date:

Purchase Again: YES   NO

INGREDIENTS:

Overall Review:

Item:

Brand: Price:

Purchase Date:

Purchase Place:

Expiration Date:

Purchase Again: YES   NO

INGREDIENTS:

Overall Review:

Product Reviews

Item:

Brand: Price:
                                Purchase Date:

Purchase Place:

Expiration Date:

Purchase Again: YES   NO

INGREDIENTS:

Overall Review:

Item:

Brand: Price:
                                Purchase Date:

Purchase Place:

Expiration Date:

Purchase Again: YES   NO

INGREDIENTS:

Overall Review:

My Beauty Recipes

Name of Recipe:

_____

Used for:

_____

Ingredients:

_____

_____

_____

How to Make:

_____

_____

_____

_____

Name of Recipe:

_____

Used for:

_____

Ingredients:

_____

_____

_____

How to Make:

_____

_____

_____

_____

My Beauty Recipes

Name of Recipe:
_____

Used for:

_____

Ingredients: _____

_____

_____

How to Make: _____

_____

_____

_____

_____

Name of Recipe:
_____

Used for:

_____

Ingredients: _____

_____

_____

How to Make: _____

_____

_____

_____

My Beauty Recipes

Name of Recipe:
_____

Used for:
_____

Ingredients:
_____
_____
_____

How to Make:
_____
_____
_____
_____

Name of Recipe:
_____

Used for:
_____

Ingredients:
_____
_____
_____

How to Make:
_____
_____
_____
_____

My Beauty Recipes

Name of Recipe:

_____

Used for:

_____

Ingredients:

_____

_____

_____

How to Make:

_____

_____

_____

_____

Name of Recipe:

_____

Used for:

_____

Ingredients:

_____

_____

_____

How to Make:

_____

_____

_____

_____

My Beauty Recipes

Name of Recipe:

_____

Used for:

_____

Ingredients:

_____

_____

_____

How to Make:

_____

_____

_____

_____

Name of Recipe:

_____

Used for:

_____

Ingredients:

_____

_____

_____

How to Make:

_____

_____

_____

My Beauty Recipes

Name of Recipe:

_____

Used for:

_____

Ingredients:

_____

_____

_____

How to Make:

_____

_____

_____

_____

Name of Recipe:

_____

Used for:

_____

Ingredients:

_____

_____

_____

How to Make:

_____

_____

_____

_____

My Beauty Recipes

Name of Recipe:

_____

Used for:

_____

Ingredients:

_____

_____

_____

How to Make:

_____

_____

_____

_____

Name of Recipe:

_____

Used for:

_____

Ingredients:

_____

_____

_____

How to Make:

_____

_____

_____

_____

My Beauty Recipes

Name of Recipe:
_____

Used for:
_____

Ingredients:
_____

_____

_____

How to Make:
_____

_____

_____

_____

Name of Recipe:
_____

Used for:
_____

Ingredients:
_____

_____

_____

How to Make:
_____

_____

_____

_____

My Beauty Recipes

Name of Recipe:

_____

Used for:

_____

Ingredients:

_____

_____

_____

How to Make:

_____

_____

_____

_____

Name of Recipe:

_____

Used for:

_____

Ingredients:

_____

_____

_____

How to Make:

_____

_____

_____

_____

My Beauty Recipes

Name of Recipe:

_____

Used for:

_____

Ingredients:

_____

_____

_____

How to Make:

_____

_____

_____

_____

Name of Recipe:

_____

Used for:

_____

Ingredients:

_____

_____

_____

How to Make:

_____

_____

_____

_____

My Beauty Journal

Date:
_____

Beauty Steps:
_____
1. _____
2. _____
3. _____
4. _____
5. _____

Hair & Body Care

_____
_____
_____

I Feel Beautiful Today Because

_____
_____
_____

Sleep Tracker (Hours slept)

1   2   3   4   5   6   7   8   9   10   11   12

Water Intake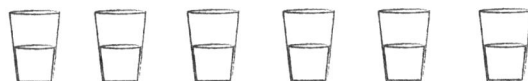

My Beauty Journal

Date:
_____

Beauty Steps:
_____

1. _____
2. _____
3. _____
4. _____
5. _____

Hair & Body Care

_____

_____

_____

_____

I Feel Beautiful Today Because

_____

_____

_____

_____

Sleep Tracker (Hours slept)

1   2   3   4   5   6   7   8   9   10   11   12

Water Intake

My Beauty Journal

Date:

_____

Beauty Steps:

_____

1. _____

2. _____

3. _____

4. _____

5. _____

Hair & Body Care

_____

_____

_____

_____

I Feel Beautiful Today Because

_____

_____

_____

_____

Sleep Tracker (Hours slept)

1   2   3   4   5   6   7   8   9   10   11   12

Water Intake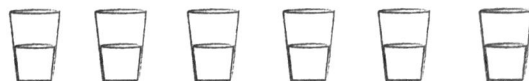

My Beauty Journal

Date:
_____

Beauty Steps:
_____
1. _____
2. _____
3. _____
4. _____
5. _____

Hair & Body Care

_____

_____

_____

I Feel Beautiful Today Because

_____

_____

_____

Sleep Tracker (Hours slept)

1   2   3   4   5   6   7   8   9   10   11   12

Water Intake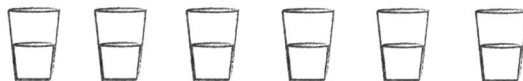

My Beauty Journal

Date:

_____

Beauty Steps:

_____

1. _____

2. _____

3. _____

4. _____

5. _____

Hair & Body Care

_____

_____

_____

I Feel Beautiful Today Because

_____

_____

_____

Sleep Tracker (Hours slept)

1   2   3   4   5   6   7   8   9   10   11   12

Water Intake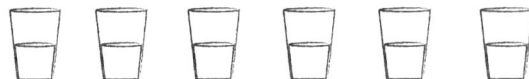

My Beauty Journal

Date:

_____

Beauty Steps:

_____

1. _____

2. _____

3. _____

4. _____

5. _____

Hair & Body Care

_____

_____

_____

I Feel Beautiful Today Because

_____

_____

_____

Sleep Tracker (Hours slept)

1 2 3 4 5 6 7 8 9 10 11 12

Water Intake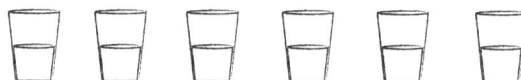

My Beauty Journal

Date:
_____

Beauty Steps:
_____
1. _____
2. _____
3. _____
4. _____
5. _____

Hair & Body Care

_____

_____

_____

I Feel Beautiful Today Because

_____

_____

_____

Sleep Tracker (Hours slept)

1   2   3   4   5   6   7   8   9   10   11   12

Water Intake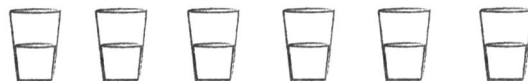

My Beauty Journal

Date:

Beauty Steps:

1.
2.
3.
4.
5.

Hair & Body Care

I Feel Beautiful Today Because

Sleep Tracker (Hours slept)

1   2   3   4   5   6   7   8   9   10   11   12

Water Intake

My Beauty Journal

Date:

_____

Beauty Steps:

_____

1. _____

2. _____

3. _____

4. _____

5. _____

Hair & Body Care

_____

_____

_____

I Feel Beautiful Today Because

_____

_____

_____

Sleep Tracker (Hours slept)

1   2   3   4   5   6   7   8   9   10   11   12

Water Intake

My Beauty Journal

Date:
_____

Beauty Steps:
_____
1. _____
2. _____
3. _____
4. _____
5. _____

Hair & Body Care

_____

_____

_____

I Feel Beautiful Today Because

_____

_____

_____

Sleep Tracker (Hours slept)

1   2   3   4   5   6   7   8   9   10   11   12

Water Intake

My Beauty Journal

Date:

_____

Beauty Steps:

_____

1. _____
2. _____
3. _____
4. _____
5. _____

Hair & Body Care

_____

_____

_____

I Feel Beautiful Today Because

_____

_____

_____

Sleep Tracker (Hours slept)

   1 2 3 4 5 6 7 8 9 10 11 12

Water Intake

My Beauty Journal

Date:
_____

Beauty Steps:
_____

1. _____

2. _____

3. _____

4. _____

5. _____

Hair & Body Care

_____

_____

_____

I Feel Beautiful Today Because

_____

_____

_____

Sleep Tracker (Hours slept)

1   2   3   4   5   6   7   8   9   10   11   12

Water Intake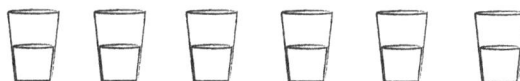

My Beauty Journal

Date:
_____

Beauty Steps:
_____
1. _____
2. _____
3. _____
4. _____
5. _____

Hair & Body Care

_____
_____
_____
_____

I Feel Beautiful Today Because

_____
_____
_____
_____

Sleep Tracker (Hours slept)

1   2   3   4   5   6   7   8   9   10   11   12

Water Intake

My Beauty Journal

Date:
_____

Beauty Steps:
_____
1. _____
2. _____
3. _____
4. _____
5. _____

Hair & Body Care

_____
_____
_____
_____

I Feel Beautiful Today Because

_____
_____
_____
_____

Sleep Tracker (Hours slept)

1 2 3 4 5 6 7 8 9 10 11 12

Water Intake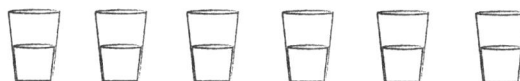

My Beauty Journal

Date:

_____

Beauty Steps:

_____
1. _____
2. _____
3. _____
4. _____
5. _____

Hair & Body Care

_____

_____

_____

_____

I Feel Beautiful Today Because

_____

_____

_____

_____

Sleep Tracker (Hours slept)

1   2   3   4   5   6   7   8   9   10   11   12

Water Intake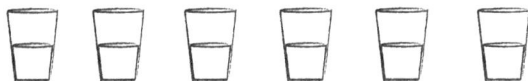

My Beauty Journal

Date:

Beauty Steps:

1.

2.

3.

4.

5.

Hair & Body Care

I Feel Beautiful Today Because

Sleep Tracker (Hours slept)

1 2 3 4 5 6 7 8 9 10 11 12

Water Intake

My Beauty Journal

Date:

_____

Beauty Steps:

_____
1. _____
2. _____
3. _____
4. _____
5. _____

Hair & Body Care

_____

_____

_____

I Feel Beautiful Today Because

_____

_____

_____

Sleep Tracker (Hours slept)

1 2 3 4 5 6 7 8 9 10 11 12

Water Intake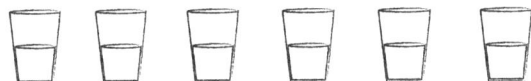

My Beauty Journal

Date:
_____

Beauty Steps:
_____
1. _____
2. _____
3. _____
4. _____
5. _____

Hair & Body Care

_____

_____

_____

I Feel Beautiful Today Because

_____

_____

_____

Sleep Tracker (Hours slept)

1   2   3   4   5   6   7   8   9   10   11   12

Water Intake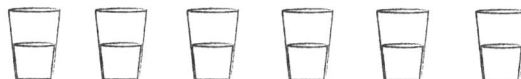

My Beauty Journal

Date:

_____

Beauty Steps:

_____
1. _____
2. _____
3. _____
4. _____
5. _____

Hair & Body Care

_____

_____

_____

I Feel Beautiful Today Because

_____

_____

_____

Sleep Tracker (Hours slept)

1 2 3 4 5 6 7 8 9 10 11 12

Water Intake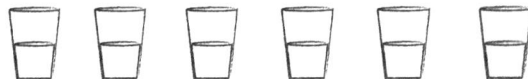

My Beauty Journal

Date:

Beauty Steps:

1.
2.
3.
4.
5.

Hair & Body Care

I Feel Beautiful Today Because

Sleep Tracker (Hours slept)

1 2 3 4 5 6 7 8 9 10 11 12

Water Intake

My Beauty Journal

Date:

_____

Beauty Steps:

_____

1. _____

2. _____

3. _____

4. _____

5. _____

Hair & Body Care

_____

_____

_____

I Feel Beautiful Today Because

_____

_____

_____

Sleep Tracker (Hours slept)

1   2   3   4   5   6   7   8   9   10   11   12

Water Intake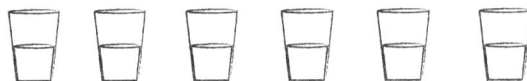

My Beauty Journal

Date:

_____

Beauty Steps:

_____

1. _____
2. _____
3. _____
4. _____
5. _____

Hair & Body Care

_____

_____

_____

I Feel Beautiful Today Because

_____

_____

_____

Sleep Tracker (Hours slept)

1 2 3 4 5 6 7 8 9 10 11 12

Water Intake

My Beauty Journal

Date:

_____

Beauty Steps:
_____
1. _____
2. _____
3. _____
4. _____
5. _____

Hair & Body Care

_____

_____

_____

I Feel Beautiful Today Because

_____

_____

_____

Sleep Tracker (Hours slept)

1   2   3   4   5   6   7   8   9   10   11   12

Water Intake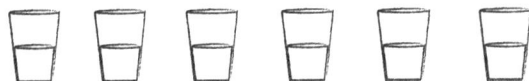

My Beauty Journal

Date:

_____

Beauty Steps:

_____

1. _____

2. _____

3. _____

4. _____

5. _____

Hair & Body Care

_____

_____

_____

_____

I Feel Beautiful Today Because

_____

_____

_____

_____

Sleep Tracker (Hours slept)

1 2 3 4 5 6 7 8 9 10 11 12

Water Intake

My Beauty Journal

Date:
_____

Beauty Steps:
_____
1. _____
2. _____
3. _____
4. _____
5. _____

Hair & Body Care

_____
_____
_____

I Feel Beautiful Today Because

_____
_____
_____

Sleep Tracker (Hours slept)

1   2   3   4   5   6   7   8   9   10   11   12

Water Intake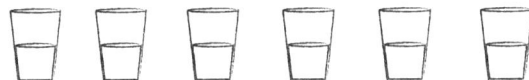

My Beauty Journal

Date:

_____

Beauty Steps:

_____

1. _____

2. _____

3. _____

4. _____

5. _____

Hair & Body Care

_____

_____

_____

I Feel Beautiful Today Because

_____

_____

_____

Sleep Tracker (Hours slept)

1   2   3   4   5   6   7   8   9   10   11   12

Water Intake

My Beauty Journal

Date:

_____

Beauty Steps:

_____

1. _____

2. _____

3. _____

4. _____

5. _____

Hair & Body Care

_____

_____

_____

I Feel Beautiful Today Because

_____

_____

_____

Sleep Tracker (Hours slept)

1 2 3 4 5 6 7 8 9 10 11 12

Water Intake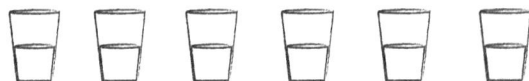

My Beauty Journal

Date:
_____

Beauty Steps:
_____

1. _____
2. _____
3. _____
4. _____
5. _____

Hair & Body Care

_____

_____

_____

I Feel Beautiful Today Because

_____

_____

_____

Sleep Tracker (Hours slept)

1   2   3   4   5   6   7   8   9   10   11   12

Water Intake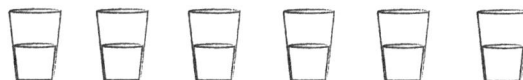

My Beauty Journal

Date:

_____

Beauty Steps:

_____

1. _____
2. _____
3. _____
4. _____
5. _____

Hair & Body Care

_____

_____

_____

_____

I Feel Beautiful Today Because

_____

_____

_____

_____

Sleep Tracker (Hours slept)

1 2 3 4 5 6 7 8 9 10 11 12

Water Intake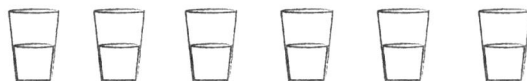

My Beauty Journal

Date:
_____

Beauty Steps:
_____

1. _____
2. _____
3. _____
4. _____
5. _____

Hair & Body Care

_____

_____

_____

I Feel Beautiful Today Because

_____

_____

_____

Sleep Tracker (Hours slept)

1 2 3 4 5 6 7 8 9 10 11 12

Water Intake

My Beauty Journal

Date:

_____

Beauty Steps:

_____

1. _____

2. _____

3. _____

4. _____

5. _____

Hair & Body Care

_____

_____

_____

I Feel Beautiful Today Because

_____

_____

_____

Sleep Tracker (Hours slept)

1   2   3   4   5   6   7   8   9   10   11   12

Water Intake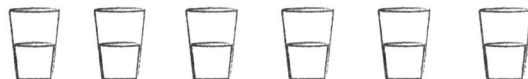

My Beauty Journal

Date:
_____

Beauty Steps:
_____

1. _____
2. _____
3. _____
4. _____
5. _____

Hair & Body Care

_____

_____

_____

I Feel Beautiful Today Because

_____

_____

_____

Sleep Tracker (Hours slept)

1 2 3 4 5 6 7 8 9 10 11 12

Water Intake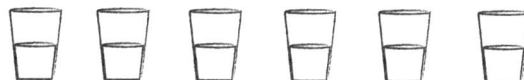

My Beauty Journal

Date:
_____

Beauty Steps:
_____
1. _____
2. _____
3. _____
4. _____
5. _____

Hair & Body Care

_____
_____
_____
_____

I Feel Beautiful Today Because

_____
_____
_____
_____

Sleep Tracker (Hours slept)

1   2   3   4   5   6   7   8   9   10   11   12

Water Intake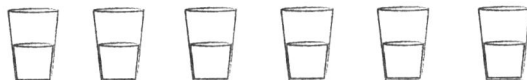

My Beauty Journal

Date:

Beauty Steps:

1.
2.
3.
4.
5.

Hair & Body Care

I Feel Beautiful Today Because

Sleep Tracker (Hours slept)

1 2 3 4 5 6 7 8 9 10 11 12

Water Intake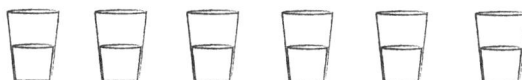

My Beauty Journal

Date:
_____

Beauty Steps:
_____
1. _____
2. _____
3. _____
4. _____
5. _____

Hair & Body Care

_____
_____
_____
_____

I Feel Beautiful Today Because

_____
_____
_____
_____

Sleep Tracker (Hours slept)

1 2 3 4 5 6 7 8 9 10 11 12

Water Intake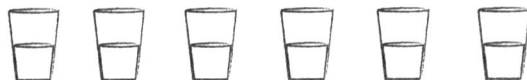

My Beauty Journal

Date:

_____

Beauty Steps:

_____

1. _____
2. _____
3. _____
4. _____
5. _____

Hair & Body Care

_____

_____

_____

_____

I Feel Beautiful Today Because

_____

_____

_____

_____

Sleep Tracker (Hours slept)

1   2   3   4   5   6   7   8   9   10   11   12

Water Intake

My Beauty Journal

Date:
_____

Beauty Steps:
_____
1. _____
2. _____
3. _____
4. _____
5. _____

Hair & Body Care

_____
_____
_____
_____

I Feel Beautiful Today Because

_____
_____
_____
_____

Sleep Tracker (Hours slept)

1   2   3   4   5   6   7   8   9   10   11   12

Water Intake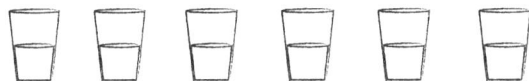

My Beauty Journal

Date:

_____

Beauty Steps:

_____

1. _____

2. _____

3. _____

4. _____

5. _____

Hair & Body Care

_____

_____

_____

I Feel Beautiful Today Because

_____

_____

_____

Sleep Tracker (Hours slept)

1 2 3 4 5 6 7 8 9 10 11 12

Water Intake

My Beauty Journal

Date:

_____

Beauty Steps:

_____

1. _____

2. _____

3. _____

4. _____

5. _____

Hair & Body Care

_____

_____

_____

I Feel Beautiful Today Because

_____

_____

_____

Sleep Tracker (Hours slept)

1   2   3   4   5   6   7   8   9   10   11   12

Water Intake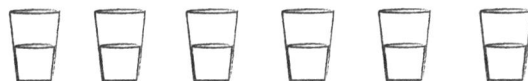

My Beauty Journal

Date:
_____

Beauty Steps:
_____
1. _____
2. _____
3. _____
4. _____
5. _____

Hair & Body Care

_____
_____
_____
_____

I Feel Beautiful Today Because

_____
_____
_____
_____

Sleep Tracker (Hours slept)

1   2   3   4   5   6   7   8   9   10   11   12

Water Intake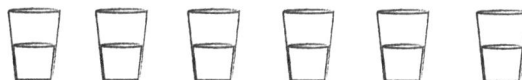

My Beauty Journal

Date:

_____

Beauty Steps:

1. _____
2. _____
3. _____
4. _____
5. _____

Hair & Body Care

_____

_____

_____

I Feel Beautiful Today Because

_____

_____

_____

Sleep Tracker (Hours slept)

1   2   3   4   5   6   7   8   9   10   11   12

Water Intake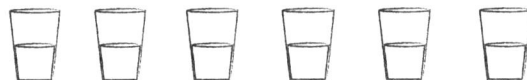

My Beauty Journal

Date:
_____

Beauty Steps:
_____

1. _____
2. _____
3. _____
4. _____
5. _____

Hair & Body Care

_____

_____

_____

I Feel Beautiful Today Because

_____

_____

_____

Sleep Tracker (Hours slept)

1   2   3   4   5   6   7   8   9   10   11   12

Water Intake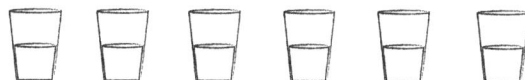

My Beauty Journal

Date:

_____

Beauty Steps:

_____

1. _____

2. _____

3. _____

4. _____

5. _____

Hair & Body Care

_____

_____

_____

I Feel Beautiful Today Because

_____

_____

_____

Sleep Tracker (Hours slept)

1 2 3 4 5 6 7 8 9 10 11 12

Water Intake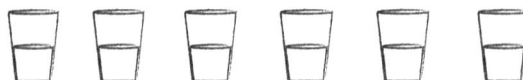

My Beauty Journal

Date:
_____

Beauty Steps:
_____
1. _____
2. _____
3. _____
4. _____
5. _____

Hair & Body Care

_____
_____
_____
_____

I Feel Beautiful Today Because

_____
_____
_____
_____

Sleep Tracker (Hours slept)

1 2 3 4 5 6 7 8 9 10 11 12

Water Intake ⬜ ⬜ ⬜ ⬜ ⬜ ⬜

My Beauty Journal

Date:

_____

Beauty Steps:

_____

1. _____

2. _____

3. _____

4. _____

5. _____

Hair & Body Care

_____

_____

_____

I Feel Beautiful Today Because

_____

_____

_____

Sleep Tracker (Hours slept)

1   2   3   4   5   6   7   8   9   10   11   12

Water Intake

My Beauty Journal

Date:

_____

Beauty Steps:

_____

1. _____
2. _____
3. _____
4. _____
5. _____

Hair & Body Care

_____

_____

_____

I Feel Beautiful Today Because

_____

_____

_____

Sleep Tracker (Hours slept)

1   2   3   4   5   6   7   8   9   10   11   12

Water Intake

My Beauty Journal

Date:
_____

Beauty Steps:
_____
1. _____
2. _____
3. _____
4. _____
5. _____

Hair & Body Care

_____

_____

_____

I Feel Beautiful Today Because

_____

_____

_____

Sleep Tracker (Hours slept)

1   2   3   4   5   6   7   8   9   10   11   12

Water Intake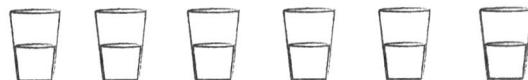

My Beauty Journal

Date:

_____

Beauty Steps:

_____

1. _____

2. _____

3. _____

4. _____

5. _____

Hair & Body Care

_____

_____

_____

_____

I Feel Beautiful Today Because

_____

_____

_____

_____

Sleep Tracker (Hours slept)

1   2   3   4   5   6   7   8   9   10   11   12

Water Intake

My Beauty Journal

Date:

Beauty Steps:

1.
2.
3.
4.
5.

Hair & Body Care

I Feel Beautiful Today Because

Sleep Tracker (Hours slept)

1 2 3 4 5 6 7 8 9 10 11 12

Water Intake

My Beauty Journal

Date:
_____

Beauty Steps:
_____

1. _____
2. _____
3. _____
4. _____
5. _____

Hair & Body Care

_____

_____

_____

I Feel Beautiful Today Because

_____

_____

_____

Sleep Tracker (Hours slept)

1 2 3 4 5 6 7 8 9 10 11 12

Water Intake

My Beauty Journal

Date:
_____

Beauty Steps:
_____
1. _____
2. _____
3. _____
4. _____
5. _____

Hair & Body Care

_____
_____
_____

I Feel Beautiful Today Because

_____
_____
_____

Sleep Tracker (Hours slept)

1 2 3 4 5 6 7 8 9 10 11 12

Water Intake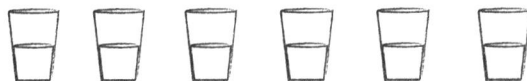

My Beauty Journal

Date:

_____

Beauty Steps:

_____

1. _____

2. _____

3. _____

4. _____

5. _____

Hair & Body Care

_____

_____

_____

_____

I Feel Beautiful Today Because

_____

_____

_____

_____

Sleep Tracker (Hours slept)

1 2 3 4 5 6 7 8 9 10 11 12

Water Intake

My Beauty Journal

Date:
_____

Beauty Steps:
_____
1. _____
2. _____
3. _____
4. _____
5. _____

Hair & Body Care

_____
_____
_____
_____

I Feel Beautiful Today Because

_____
_____
_____
_____

Sleep Tracker (Hours slept)

1 2 3 4 5 6 7 8 9 10 11 12

Water Intake

My Beauty Journal

Date:

Beauty Steps:

1.
2.
3.
4.
5.

Hair & Body Care

I Feel Beautiful Today Because

Sleep Tracker (Hours slept)

1 2 3 4 5 6 7 8 9 10 11 12

Water Intake

My Beauty Journal

Date:
_____

Beauty Steps:
_____
1. _____
2. _____
3. _____
4. _____
5. _____

Hair & Body Care

_____

_____

_____

I Feel Beautiful Today Because

_____

_____

_____

Sleep Tracker (Hours slept)

1   2   3   4   5   6   7   8   9   10   11   12

Water Intake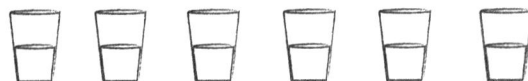

My Beauty Journal

Date:

_____

Beauty Steps:

_____

1. _____

2. _____

3. _____

4. _____

5. _____

Hair & Body Care

_____

_____

_____

_____

I Feel Beautiful Today Because

_____

_____

_____

_____

Sleep Tracker (Hours slept)

1   2   3   4   5   6   7   8   9   10   11   12

Water Intake

My Beauty Journal

Date:

_____

Beauty Steps:

_____

1. _____

2. _____

3. _____

4. _____

5. _____

Hair & Body Care

_____

_____

_____

I Feel Beautiful Today Because

_____

_____

_____

Sleep Tracker (Hours slept)

1   2   3   4   5   6   7   8   9   10   11   12

Water Intake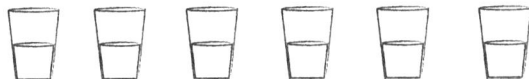

My Beauty Journal

Date:

_____

Beauty Steps:

_____

1. _____

2. _____

3. _____

4. _____

5. _____

Hair & Body Care

_____

_____

_____

_____

I Feel Beautiful Today Because

_____

_____

_____

_____

Sleep Tracker (Hours slept)

1   2   3   4   5   6   7   8   9   10   11   12

Water Intake

My Beauty Journal

Date:
_____

Beauty Steps:
_____
1. _____
2. _____
3. _____
4. _____
5. _____

Hair & Body Care

_____
_____
_____
_____

I Feel Beautiful Today Because

_____
_____
_____
_____

Sleep Tracker (Hours slept)

1   2   3   4   5   6   7   8   9   10   11   12

Water Intake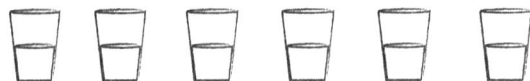

My Beauty Journal

Date:

_____

Beauty Steps:

_____

1. _____
2. _____
3. _____
4. _____
5. _____

Hair & Body Care

_____

_____

_____

I Feel Beautiful Today Because

_____

_____

_____

Sleep Tracker (Hours slept)

1   2   3   4   5   6   7   8   9   10   11   12

Water Intake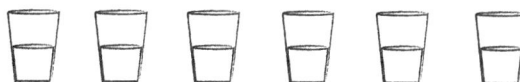

My Beauty Journal

Date:

_____

Beauty Steps:

_____

1. _____

2. _____

3. _____

4. _____

5. _____

Hair & Body Care

_____

_____

_____

I Feel Beautiful Today Because

_____

_____

_____

Sleep Tracker (Hours slept)

1   2   3   4   5   6   7   8   9   10   11   12

Water Intake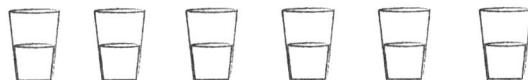

My Beauty Journal

Date:

Beauty Steps:

1.
2.
3.
4.
5.

Hair & Body Care

I Feel Beautiful Today Because

Sleep Tracker (Hours slept)

1   2   3   4   5   6   7   8   9   10   11   12

Water Intake

My Beauty Journal

Date:

_____

Beauty Steps:

_____

1. _____

2. _____

3. _____

4. _____

5. _____

Hair & Body Care

_____

_____

_____

I Feel Beautiful Today Because

_____

_____

_____

Sleep Tracker (Hours slept)

1 2 3 4 5 6 7 8 9 10 11 12

Water Intake

My Beauty Journal

Date:
_____

Beauty Steps:
_____
1. _____
2. _____
3. _____
4. _____
5. _____

Hair & Body Care

_____
_____
_____
_____

I Feel Beautiful Today Because

_____
_____
_____

Sleep Tracker (Hours slept)

1   2   3   4   5   6   7   8   9   10   11   12

Water Intake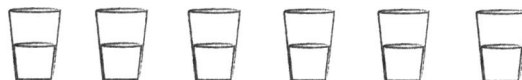

My Beauty Journal

Date:
_____

Beauty Steps:
_____
1. _____
2. _____
3. _____
4. _____
5. _____

Hair & Body Care

_____
_____
_____

I Feel Beautiful Today Because

_____
_____
_____

Sleep Tracker (Hours slept)

1 2 3 4 5 6 7 8 9 10 11 12

Water Intake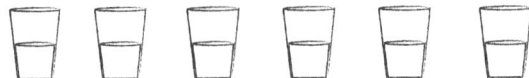

My Beauty Journal

Date:

_____

Beauty Steps:

_____

1. _____

2. _____

3. _____

4. _____

5. _____

Hair & Body Care

_____

_____

_____

_____

I Feel Beautiful Today Because

_____

_____

_____

Sleep Tracker (Hours slept)

1 2 3 4 5 6 7 8 9 10 11 12

Water Intake

My Beauty Journal

Date:

_____

Beauty Steps:

_____

1. _____
2. _____
3. _____
4. _____
5. _____

Hair & Body Care

_____

_____

_____

_____

I Feel Beautiful Today Because

_____

_____

_____

_____

Sleep Tracker (Hours slept)

1   2   3   4   5   6   7   8   9   10   11   12

Water Intake

My Beauty Journal

Date:
_____

Beauty Steps:
_____
1. _____
2. _____
3. _____
4. _____
5. _____

Hair & Body Care

_____
_____
_____

I Feel Beautiful Today Because

_____
_____
_____

Sleep Tracker (Hours slept)

1   2   3   4   5   6   7   8   9   10   11   12

Water Intake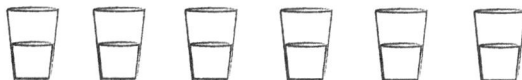

My Beauty Journal

Date:
_____

Beauty Steps:
_____
1. _____
2. _____
3. _____
4. _____
5. _____

Hair & Body Care

_____

_____

_____

I Feel Beautiful Today Because

_____

_____

_____

Sleep Tracker (Hours slept)

1 2 3 4 5 6 7 8 9 10 11 12

Water Intake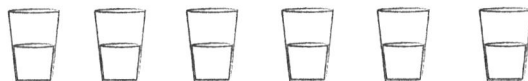

My Beauty Journal

Date:
_____

Beauty Steps:
_____
1. _____
2. _____
3. _____
4. _____
5. _____

Hair & Body Care

_____
_____
_____
_____

I Feel Beautiful Today Because

_____
_____
_____
_____

Sleep Tracker (Hours slept)

1 2 3 4 5 6 7 8 9 10 11 12

Water Intake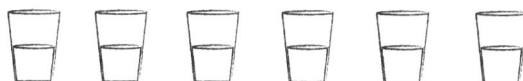

My Beauty Journal

Date:

_____

Beauty Steps:

_____

1. _____

2. _____

3. _____

4. _____

5. _____

Hair & Body Care

_____

_____

_____

_____

I Feel Beautiful Today Because

_____

_____

_____

_____

Sleep Tracker (Hours slept)

1   2   3   4   5   6   7   8   9   10   11   12

Water Intake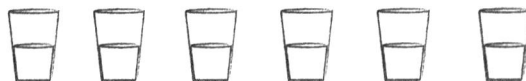

My Beauty Journal

Date:
_____

Beauty Steps:
_____

1. _____
2. _____
3. _____
4. _____
5. _____

Hair & Body Care

_____

_____

_____

_____

I Feel Beautiful Today Because

_____

_____

_____

_____

Sleep Tracker (Hours slept)

1   2   3   4   5   6   7   8   9   10   11   12

Water Intake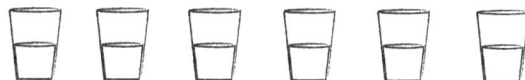

My Beauty Journal

Date:

_____

Beauty Steps:

_____

1. _____
2. _____
3. _____
4. _____
5. _____

Hair & Body Care

_____

_____

_____

I Feel Beautiful Today Because

_____

_____

_____

Sleep Tracker (Hours slept)

1 2 3 4 5 6 7 8 9 10 11 12

Water Intake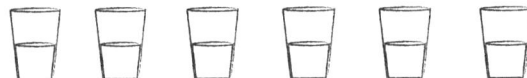

My Beauty Journal

Date:

_____

Beauty Steps:

_____

1. _____
2. _____
3. _____
4. _____
5. _____

Hair & Body Care

_____

_____

_____

I Feel Beautiful Today Because

_____

_____

_____

Sleep Tracker (Hours slept)

1 2 3 4 5 6 7 8 9 10 11 12

Water Intake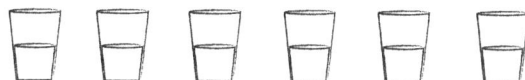

My Beauty Journal

Date:
_____

Beauty Steps:
_____
1. _____
2. _____
3. _____
4. _____
5. _____

Hair & Body Care

_____
_____
_____
_____

I Feel Beautiful Today Because

_____
_____
_____
_____

Sleep Tracker (Hours slept)

1 2 3 4 5 6 7 8 9 10 11 12

Water Intake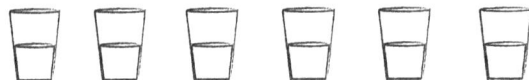

My Beauty Journal

Date:

Beauty Steps:

1.
2.
3.
4.
5.

Hair & Body Care

I Feel Beautiful Today Because

Sleep Tracker (Hours slept)

1   2   3   4   5   6   7   8   9   10   11   12

Water Intake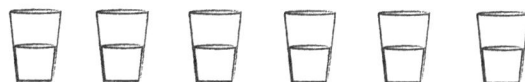

My Beauty Journal

Date:
_____

Beauty Steps:
_____
1. _____
2. _____
3. _____
4. _____
5. _____

Hair & Body Care

_____
_____
_____
_____

I Feel Beautiful Today Because

_____
_____
_____
_____

Sleep Tracker (Hours slept)

   1   2   3   4   5   6   7   8   9   10   11   12

Water Intake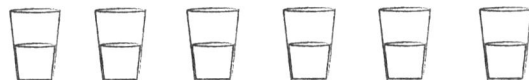

My Beauty Journal

Date:

Beauty Steps:

1.

2.

3.

4.

5.

Hair & Body Care

I Feel Beautiful Today Because

Sleep Tracker (Hours slept)

1 2 3 4 5 6 7 8 9 10 11 12

Water Intake

My Beauty Journal

Date:

_____

Beauty Steps:

_____

1. _____

2. _____

3. _____

4. _____

5. _____

Hair & Body Care

_____

_____

_____

I Feel Beautiful Today Because

_____

_____

_____

Sleep Tracker (Hours slept)

1 2 3 4 5 6 7 8 9 10 11 12

Water Intake

www.ingramcontent.com/pod-product-compliance
Lightning Source LLC
Chambersburg PA
CBHW080600030426
42336CB00019B/3274